THE COMPLETE INTERSTITIAL CYSTITIS DIET COOKBOOK FOR BEGINNERS

A Personalized Diet Plan for IC Management, Reducing Bladder Irritation, Easing Pelvic Pains, and Frequency of Urination

Dr. Anna Fennell

COPYRIGHT

TABLE OF CONTENTS

CHAPTER ONE

INTRODUCTION TO INTERSTITIAL CYSTITIS (IC)

Interstitial cystitis is a chronic condition causing bladder pressure, bladder pain and sometimes pelvic pain. The pain ranges from mild discomfort to severe pain. The condition is a part of a spectrum of diseases known as painful bladder syndrome.

Your bladder is a hollow, muscular organ that stores urine. The bladder expands until it's full and then signals your brain that it's time to urinate, communicating through the pelvic nerves. This creates the urge to urinate for most people.

Causes and Risk Factors

Causes

The exact cause of interstitial cystitis isn't known, but it's likely that many factors contribute. For instance, people with interstitial cystitis may also have a defect in the protective lining (epithelium) of the bladder. A leak in the epithelium may allow toxic substances in urine to irritate your bladder wall.

Other possible but unproven contributing factors include an autoimmune reaction, heredity, infection or allergy.

Risk factors

These factors are associated with a higher risk of interstitial cystitis:

Your sex: Women are diagnosed with interstitial cystitis more often than men. Symptoms in men may mimic interstitial cystitis, but they're more often associated with an inflammation of the prostate gland (prostatitis).

Your age: Most people with interstitial cystitis are diagnosed during their 30s or older.

Having a chronic pain disorder: Interstitial cystitis may be associated with other chronic pain disorder, such as irritable bowel syndrome or fibromyalgia.

Complications

Interstitial cystitis can result in a number of complications, including:

Reduced bladder capacity: Interstitial cystitis can cause stiffening of the bladder wall, which allows your bladder to hold less urine.

Lower quality of life: Frequent urination and pain may interfere with social activities, work and other activities of daily life.

Sexual intimacy problems: Frequent urination and pain may strain your personal relationships, and sexual intimacy may suffer.

Emotional troubles: The chronic pain and interrupted sleep associated with interstitial cystitis may cause emotional stress and can lead to depression.

Symptoms and Diagnosis

Symptoms

The signs and symptoms of interstitial cystitis vary from person to person. If you have interstitial cystitis, your symptoms may also vary over time, periodically flaring in response to common triggers, such as menstruation, sitting for a long time, stress, exercise and sexual activity.

Interstitial cystitis signs and symptoms include:

Pain in your pelvis or between the vagina and anus in women

Pain between the scrotum and anus (perineum) in men

Chronic pelvic pain

A persistent, urgent need to urinate

Frequent urination, often of small amounts, throughout the day and night (up to 60 times a day)

Pain or discomfort while the bladder fills and relief after urinating

Pain during sex

Symptoms severity is different for everyone, and some people may experience symptom-free periods.

Although signs and symptoms of interstitial cystitis may resemble those of a chronic urinary tract infection, there's usually no infection. However, symptoms may worsen if a person with interstitial cystitis gets a urinary tract infection.

Your bladder, kidneys, ureters and urethra make up your urinary system. When you have interstitial cystitis, the walls of your bladder become irritated and inflamed, compared with those of a normal bladder.

With interstitial cystitis, these signals get mixed up — you feel the need to urinate more often and with smaller volumes of urine than most people.

Interstitial cystitis most often affects women and can have a long-lasting impact on quality of life. Although there's no cure, medications and other therapies may offer relief

Diagnosis

Diagnosis of interstitial cystitis might include:

Medical history and bladder diary: Your health care provider may ask you to describe your symptoms and to keep a bladder diary, recording the volume of fluids you drink and the volume of urine you pass.

Pelvic exam: During a pelvic exam, your provider examines your external genitals, vagina and cervix and feels your abdomen to assess your internal pelvic organs. Your provider may also examine your anus and rectum.

Urine test: A sample of your urine is analyzed for signs of a urinary tract infection.

Cystoscopy: Your provider inserts a thin tube with a tiny camera (cystoscope) through the urethra, showing the lining of your bladder. Your provider may also inject liquid into your bladder to measure your bladder capacity. Your provider may perform this procedure, known as hydrodistention, after you've been numbed with an anesthetic medication to make you more comfortable.

Biopsy: During cystoscopy under anesthesia, your provider may remove a sample of tissue (biopsy) from the bladder and the urethra for examination under a microscope. This is to check for bladder cancer and other rare causes of bladder pain.

Urine cytology: Your provider collects a urine sample and examines the cells to help rule out cancer.

Potassium sensitivity test: Your provider places (instills) two solutions — water and potassium chloride — into your bladder, one at a time. You're asked to rate on a scale of 0 to 5 the pain and urgency you feel after each solution is instilled. If you feel noticeably more pain or urgency with the potassium solution than with the water, your provider may diagnose interstitial cystitis. People with typical bladders can't tell the difference between the two solutions.

Treatment and Management

No simple treatment eliminates the signs and symptoms of interstitial cystitis, and no one treatment works for everyone. You may need to try various treatments or combinations of treatments before you find an approach that relieves your symptoms.

Physical therapy

Working with a physical therapist may relieve pelvic pain associated with muscle tenderness, restrictive connective tissue or muscle abnormalities in your pelvic floor.

Oral medications

Certain medicines that you take by mouth (oral medications) may improve signs and symptoms of interstitial cystitis:

Nonsteroidal anti-inflammatory drugs, such as ibuprofen (Advil, Motrin IB, others) or naproxen sodium (Aleve), to relieve pain.

Tricyclic antidepressants, such as amitriptyline or imipramine (Tofranil), to help relax your bladder and block pain.

Antihistamines, such as loratadine (Claritin, others), which may reduce urinary urgency and frequency and relieve other symptoms.

Pentosan polysulfate sodium (Elmiron), which is approved by the Food and Drug Administration specifically for treating interstitial cystitis. How it works is unknown, but it may restore the inner surface of the bladder, which protects the bladder wall from substances in urine that could irritate it. It may take two to four months before you begin to feel pain relief and up to six months to experience a decrease in urinary frequency.

Macular eye disease has been associated with use of this medication in some people. Before starting this treatment, you may need a comprehensive eye exam. You may also need additional eye exams to monitor for eye disease as you continue therapy.

Nerve stimulation

Nerve stimulation techniques include:

Transcutaneous electrical nerve stimulation (TENS): With TENS, mild electrical pulses relieve pelvic pain and, in some cases, reduce urinary frequency. TENS may increase blood flow to the bladder. This may strengthen the muscles that help control the bladder or trigger the release of substances that block pain.

Electrical wires placed on your lower back or just above your pubic area deliver electrical pulses — the length of time and frequency of therapy depends on what works best for you.

Sacral nerve stimulation. Your sacral nerves are a primary link between the spinal cord and nerves in your bladder. Stimulating these nerves may reduce urinary urgency associated with interstitial cystitis.

With sacral nerve stimulation, a thin wire placed near the sacral nerves sends electrical impulses to your bladder, similar to what a pacemaker does for your heart. If the procedure decreases your symptoms, you may have a permanent device surgically implanted. This procedure doesn't manage pain from interstitial cystitis, but may help to relieve some symptoms of urinary frequency and urgency.

Sacral nerve stimulation device

During sacral nerve stimulation, a surgically implanted device delivers electrical impulses to the nerves that regulate bladder activity. These are called the sacral nerves. The unit is placed under the skin in the lower back, about where the back pocket is on a pair of pants. In this image, the device is shown out of place to allow a better view of the unit.

Bladder distention

Some people notice a temporary improvement in symptoms after cystoscopy with bladder distention. Bladder distention is the stretching of the bladder with water. If you have long-term improvement, the procedure may be repeated.

Botulinum toxin A (Botox) may be injected into the bladder wall during bladder distention. But, this treatment option could lead to not being able to empty your bladder completely when you urinate. You may need to self-catheterize — be able to insert a tube into your own bladder to drain urine — after this treatment.

Medications instilled into the bladder

In bladder instillation, your provider places the prescription medication dimethyl sulfoxide (Rimso-50) into your bladder through a thin, flexible tube (catheter) inserted through the urethra.

The solution sometimes is mixed with other medications, such as a local anesthetic, and remains in your bladder for about 15 minutes. You urinate to expel the solution.

You might receive dimethyl sulfoxide — also called DMSO — treatment weekly for six to eight weeks, and then have maintenance treatments as needed — such as every couple of weeks, for up to one year.

Another approach to bladder instillation uses a solution containing the medications lidocaine, sodium bicarbonate, and either pentosan or heparin.

Surgery

Doctors rarely use surgery to treat interstitial cystitis because removing the bladder doesn't relieve pain and can lead to other complications.

People with severe pain or those whose bladders can hold only very small volumes of urine are possible candidates for surgery, but usually only after other treatments fail and symptoms affect quality of life. Surgical options include:

Fulguration: This minimally invasive method involves insertion of instruments through the urethra to burn off ulcers that may be present with interstitial cystitis.

Resection: This is another minimally invasive method that involves insertion of instruments through the urethra to cut around any ulcers.

Bladder augmentation: In this procedure, a surgeon increases the capacity of your bladder by putting a patch of intestine on the bladder. However, this is performed only in very specific and rare instances. The procedure doesn't eliminate pain and some people need to empty their bladders with a catheter many times a day.

Self-Care

Some people with interstitial cystitis find symptom relief from these strategies:

Dietary changes: Eliminating or reducing foods in your diet that irritate your bladder may help to relieve the discomfort of interstitial cystitis.

Common bladder irritants — known as the "four Cs" — include: carbonated beverages, caffeine in all forms (including chocolate), citrus products and food containing high concentrations of vitamin C. Consider avoiding similar foods, such as tomatoes, pickled foods, alcohol and spices. Artificial sweeteners may aggravate symptoms in some people.

If you think certain foods may irritate your bladder, try eliminating them from your diet. Reintroduce them one at a time and pay attention to which, if any, worsen symptoms.

Bladder training: Bladder training involves timed urination — going to the toilet according to the clock rather than waiting for the need to go. You start by urinating at set intervals, such as every half-hour — whether you have to go or not. Then you gradually wait longer between bathroom visits.

During bladder training, you may learn to control urinary urges by using relaxation techniques, such as breathing slowly and deeply or distracting yourself with another activity.

These self-care measures also may help:

Wear loose clothing: Avoid belts or clothes that put pressure on your abdomen.

Reduce stress: Try methods such as visualization and biofeedback.

If you smoke, stop: Smoking may worsen any painful condition, and smoking contributes to bladder cancer.

Exercise: Easy stretching exercises may help reduce interstitial cystitis symptoms.

Impact of IC on Quality of Life

Coping and support

Interstitial cystitis can worsen your quality of life. Support from family and friends is important, but because the condition is a urinary problem, you may find the topic difficult to discuss.

Find a supportive health care provider who is concerned about your quality of life as well as your condition. Seek someone who will work with you to help relieve your urinary frequency, urgency and bladder pain.

You might also benefit from joining a support group. A support group can provide sympathetic listening and useful information. Ask your provider for information on support groups or see the Interstitial Cystitis Association on the web.

CHAPTER TWO

ROLE OF DIET IN MANAGING IC SYMPTOMS

Dietary management can be an effective treatment plan for interstitial cystitis. Diet alone may not improve the symptoms, but consuming certain foods and avoiding others can provide some relief.

Experts recommend avoiding potential triggers such as caffeine and citrus juices. However, trigger foods may vary for each person.

Many people with interstitial cystitis rely on alternative treatment because the condition currently has no cure. Usually, healthcare professionals will recommend specific dietary strategies and interventional therapies for people with the condition.

Dietary Triggers and Their Effects on IC Symptoms

Can diet trigger interstitial cystitis?

Studies suggest that certain foods can worsen bladder pain and some people with IC find that these foods or drinks trigger or worsen their symptoms. These trigger foods can intensify your symptoms of interstitial cystitis by changing the potassium content of urine and activating pain receptors in the bladder.

Coffee, soda, alcohol, tomatoes, hot and spicy foods, chocolate, caffeinated beverages, citrus juices and drinks, MSG, and high-acid foods can trigger IC symptoms or make them worse. Some people also note that their symptoms get worse after eating or drinking products with artificial sweeteners, or sweeteners that are not found naturally in foods and beverages.

A 2023 study that assessed diet sensitivities among people with interstitial cystitis or other pelvic pain and a control group without the condition found that:

About 70% of people in the interstitial cystitis group had more than one food sensitivity.

People with symptoms of interstitial cystitis were more sensitive to certain beverages and spicy foods than other groups.

Compared with white participants, Black participants with interstitial cystitis reported greater sensitivity to non-caffeinated and alcoholic drinks and a higher rate of urinary urgency.

Learning which foods trigger your symptoms or make them worse may take some effort. Keep a food diary and note the times you have bladder pain. For example, the diary might show that your symptom flares always happen after you eat tomatoes or oranges. If you find that certain foods make your symptoms worse, your health care professional and dietitian can help you avoid them with an eating plan. Find an expert to advise you on how to use nutrition and ingredient information on a food label. You can use this information to help you avoid eating or drinking things that trigger pain in your bladder.

Stopping certain foods and drinks—and then adding them back to what you normally eat and drink one at a time—may help you figure out which foods or drinks, if any, affect your symptoms. Talk with your health care professional about how much liquid you should drink to prevent dehydration based on your health, how active you are, and where you live. Water is the best liquid for bladder health.

Some doctors recommend taking an antacid with meals. This medicine reduces the amount of acid that gets into the urine.

Nutritional Considerations for IC Patients

A person with interstitial cystitis can include the following foods in their diet:

Certain fruits: avocados, bananas, blueberries, melons, pears, apricots, dates, prunes, and raisins

Some vegetables: asparagus, celery, bell pepper, broccoli, beets, eggplant, peas, mushrooms, and spinach

Grains: oats and rice

Proteins: beef, eggs, pork, lamb, poultry, and fish

Nuts: almonds, walnuts, cashews, macadamia nuts, and pistachios

Nut and seed butters: peanut butter, almond butter, cashew butter, and sunflower seed butter

Some dairy: cream cheese, cheddar cheese, and low fat and nonfat milk

Herbs and spices: basil, garlic, thyme, and rosemary

Beverages: water, pear juice, blueberry juice, grain-based coffee substitutes, and chamomile or peppermint tea.

IC- friendly foods will be discussed extensively in the next chapter.

CHAPTER THREE

FOODS TO INCLUDE AND AVOID IN AN IC DIET

In crafting an IC (Interstitial Cystitis) friendly diet, the focus is on minimizing foods and drinks that might irritate the bladder while incorporating options that are gentler on it. Here are some items commonly included:

Water: Adequate hydration is crucial for bladder health. Opting for water is generally recommended, though some individuals find distilled or higher pH water less bothersome.

Low-acid fruits: Citrus fruits can be problematic for some with IC, but options like pears, apples, and blueberries are often well-tolerated.

Vegetables: Non-citrus veggies such as cucumber, zucchini, carrots, and green beans are typically less likely to irritate the bladder.

Whole grains: Oats, brown rice, and quinoa provide fiber without causing significant bladder irritation compared to refined grains.

Lean proteins: Chicken, turkey, fish, and tofu are good protein sources that tend to be bladder-friendly.

Healthy fats: Incorporating sources like avocado, olive oil, and flaxseed oil adds beneficial fats to the diet without exacerbating IC symptoms.

Dairy alternatives: For those sensitive to dairy, options like almond milk, coconut milk, or lactose-free dairy products can be suitable replacements.

Herbal teas: Certain herbal teas such as chamomile or peppermint may offer soothing effects for the bladder.

Honey: As a natural sweetener, honey can be used in moderation as an alternative to sugar or artificial sweeteners, which may aggravate bladder symptoms in some individuals.

While these foods are generally considered safe for many with IC, it's essential to listen to your body and monitor how it responds to different foods. Keeping a food diary can help identify any triggers and customize your diet accordingly. Additionally, consulting with a healthcare professional or registered dietitian for personalized guidance is advisable.

Foods to avoid

Sure, here's a more natural version without the bold highlights:

In an IC (Interstitial Cystitis) friendly diet, it's often advised to steer clear of foods and drinks that are known to irritate the bladder. Here are some common culprits to consider avoiding:

Citrus fruits like oranges, lemons, limes, and grapefruits are acidic and can aggravate bladder symptoms in some individuals. Tomato-based products such as sauces, ketchup, and salsa are also acidic and may worsen IC symptoms. Spicy foods containing chili peppers, hot sauces, and spicy seasonings can irritate the bladder and exacerbate symptoms.

Caffeinated beverages like coffee, tea, cola, and energy drinks act as diuretics and may irritate the bladder. Alcohol, including beer, wine, and liquor, can also irritate the bladder and increase urinary frequency and urgency.

Carbonated beverages like sodas and sparkling water can aggravate bladder symptoms due to their carbonation. Some artificial sweeteners, like aspartame and saccharin, may irritate the bladder and worsen symptoms.

High-acid foods like vinegar, pickles, and certain condiments can be acidic and irritating to the bladder. Highly processed foods, including those high in preservatives, additives, and artificial ingredients, may exacerbate IC symptoms.

Highly spiced foods, such as curry dishes and heavily seasoned meats, can also be irritating to the bladder. Chocolate contains caffeine and other compounds that may irritate the bladder and worsen symptoms in some individuals.

Citrus juices like orange juice, lemonade, and other citrus juices are acidic and can irritate the bladder.

Remember, individual tolerances can vary, so it's essential to pay attention to how your body reacts to different foods and beverages. Keeping a food diary can help identify triggers and guide your dietary choices. Additionally, consulting with a healthcare professional or registered dietitian can provide personalized guidance and support for managing IC symptoms through diet.

Importance of Hydration in IC Management

Hydration is essential for managing Interstitial Cystitis (IC) symptoms and is a fundamental aspect of an IC-friendly diet. Here's why keeping well-hydrated matters:

Maintains Bladder Health: Ensuring proper hydration helps sustain the health of the bladder lining. Given that IC can cause inflammation and sensitivity in the bladder lining, dehydration can exacerbate these symptoms.

Dilutes Urine: Drinking ample water helps dilute urine, which can lessen the concentration of irritants in the bladder. This, in turn, can alleviate discomfort and urinary urgency associated with IC.

Flushes Toxins: Water aids in flushing toxins and bacteria out of the urinary tract, decreasing the likelihood of urinary tract infections (UTIs) that can worsen IC symptoms.

Reduces Bladder Irritation: Dehydration often leads to more concentrated urine, potentially heightening bladder irritation. Staying well-hydrated helps mitigate this discomfort.

Supports Overall Health: Hydration is integral to overall health and wellness. It facilitates proper digestion, circulation, temperature regulation, and organ function, all of which contribute to effectively managing IC symptoms.

Prevents Constipation: Sufficient water intake helps prevent constipation, which can aggravate IC symptoms by exerting pressure on the bladder.

Enhances Medication Effectiveness: Adequate hydration can boost the efficacy of medications used to manage IC symptoms. It ensures medications are adequately diluted and absorbed in the body.

Improves Mood and Energy Levels: Dehydration can lead to fatigue and mood swings, exacerbating the stress and discomfort associated with IC. Staying hydrated helps maintain energy levels and promotes overall well-being.

Incorporating ample water into your daily routine is crucial for managing IC symptoms. It's advisable to spread out fluid intake throughout the day rather than consuming large quantities at once to avoid overtaxing the bladder. Additionally, some individuals may find that certain types of water, like distilled water or water with a higher pH level, are less bothersome to their bladder. As always, it's important to heed your body's signals and adjust fluid intake based on your individual needs and preferences. If you have specific concerns about hydration and IC, consulting with a healthcare professional can provide tailored advice and recommendations.

CHAPTER FOUR

DELICIOUS RECIPES IDEAS FOR THE INTERSTITIAL CYSTITIS DIET

DELICIOUS INTERSTITIAL CYSTITIS DIET BREAKFAST RECIPES

Buckwheat pancakes

Ingredients

150g plain flour

150g buckwheat flour

2 tbsp caster sugar

1 tsp baking powder

1 tsp bicarbonate of soda

50g butter, melted

2 large eggs

400ml buttermilk

vegetable oil, for frying

To serve

blueberries

maple syrup

Directions

STEP 1

Combine the plain flour, buckwheat flour, sugar, ½ tsp salt, baking powder and bicarbonate of soda in a large bowl. Combine the melted butter, eggs and buttermilk in a jug and whisk to combine. Stir the wet Ingredients slowly into the dry Ingredients until combined, to make a thick batter.

STEP 2

Heat a large non-stick pan or skillet over medium heat and brush with a light layer of vegetable oil. Add a few heaped tablespoons of the mixture into the pan and form into a circle. If your pan is large enough you can do 2-3 at a time, just don't overcrowd the pan too. Once the edges are set and bubbles appear on the surface (around 2-3 mins) flip and cook for a further 2 mins. The pancakes should be a deep golden brown on both sides.

Transfer to a warm oven on low and repeat the process until the batter is all used.

STEP 3

Serve stacked with fresh blueberries and maple syrup drizzled generously over the top.

Green goddess smoothie bowl

Ingredients

2 bananas, sliced

1 ripe avocado, stoned, peeled and chopped into chunks

1 small ripe mango, stoned, peeled and chopped into chunks

100g spinach (fresh or frozen)

250ml milk (unsweetened almond or coconut milk
works well)

1 tbsp unsweetened almond or peanut butter

1 tbsp clear honey, agave or maple syrup (optional)

For the seed mix

1 tbsp chia seeds

1 tbsp linseeds

4 tbsp pumpkin seeds

4 tbsp sunflower seeds

4 tbsp coconut flakes

4 tbsp flaked almonds

¼ tsp ground cinnamon

2 tbsp clear honey, agave or maple syrup

To serve

175g mixed fresh fruit, chopped (we used banana, mango, raspberries and blueberries)

Directions

STEP 1

Slice the bananas and arrange over a small baking tray lined with parchment. Freeze for 2 hrs until solid. (You can now transfer the banana slices to a freezer bag and freeze for 3 months, or continue with the recipe.)

STEP 2

For the seed mix, heat oven to 180C/160C fan/gas 4 and line a baking tray with parchment. Tip the seeds, coconut and almonds into a bowl, add the cinnamon and drizzle over the honey, agave or maple syrup. Toss until everything is well coated, then scatter over the baking tray in an even layer. Bake for 10-15 mins, stirring every 5 mins or so, until the seeds are lightly toasted. Leave to cool. Will keep in an airtight container for up to 1 month.

STEP 3

Put the avocado, mango, spinach, milk, nut butter, frozen banana slices and honey (if using) in a blender and whizz to a thick smoothie consistency – you may have to scrape down the sides with a spoon a few times. Divide between two bowls and arrange the fruit on top. Scatter 1-2 tbsp of the seed mix over each bowl and eat straight away.

One-cup pancakes

Ingredients

1 cup plain flour

1½ cups milk

1 large egg or 2 medium eggs

20g butter

2 tbsp vegetable or sunflower oil

caster sugar and lemon wedges, to serve (optional)

Directions

STEP 1

Tip the flour and a pinch of salt into a bowl. Make a well in the centre and pour in the milk and egg. Whisk together, starting in the middle, to create a smooth batter. It should be the thickness of double cream.

STEP 2

Heat a little of the butter and oil in a non-stick frying pan. Add a sixth of the batter to the pan, quickly swirling it so there are no holes. Fry on one side for 1-2 mins then flip over and cook for a further 1 min. Keep on a plate, covered, in a warm oven. Repeat with the remaining batter to make six pancakes in total. Serve with sugar and lemon, if you like.

Maple-glazed blueberry muffins

Ingredients

250g plain flour

1 ½ tsp baking powder

1 tsp bicarbonate of soda

140g granulated sugar

100g unsalted butter, melted

50g buttermilk

2 large eggs

50g maple syrup, plus 11/2 tbsp for the topping

1 tsp vanilla extract

175g blueberries, plus extra for the top

3 tbsp icing sugar

Directions

STEP 1

Heat oven to 180C/160C fan/gas 4. Place the muffin cases in a muffin tray. In a large bowl, combine the flour, baking powder, bicarb, sugar and 1/2 tsp salt. Whisk the butter, buttermilk, eggs, maple syrup and vanilla extract in a jug. Pour the wet Ingredients into the dry and add most of the blueberries. Stir briefly to just combine, but don't overmix or the muffins will be heavy.

STEP 2

Divide the mixture between the muffin cases (use an ice cream scoop if you have one) and bake for 22-25 mins until well risen and a skewer inserted into the centre comes out clean. Transfer to a wire rack.

STEP 3

Mix the remaining maple syrup and the icing sugar together with a pinch of salt until smooth. Brush the icing over each muffin while they are still warm. Dot a few blueberries on top of each one. Best eaten within a day or two.

Cinnamon porridge with banana & berries

Ingredients

100g porridge oats

½ tsp cinnamon, plus extra to serve

4 tsp demerara sugar

450ml skimmed milk

3 bananas, sliced

400g punnet strawberries, hulled and halved

150g pot fat-free natural yogurt

Directions

STEP 1

In a medium-sized saucepan, mix the oats, cinnamon, sugar, milk and half the sliced bananas. Bring to the boil, stirring occasionally. Turn down the heat and cook for 4-5 mins, stirring all the time.

STEP 2

Remove and divide between 4 bowls, top with the remaining banana, strawberries, a dollop of yogurt and a sprinkle of cinnamon.

Peanut butter pancakes

Ingredients

250g crunchy peanut butter

50g unsalted butter, cubed, plus extra for cooking

6 tbsp maple syrup

300g self-raising flour

1 tsp baking powder

1 tbsp golden caster sugar

2 large eggs

350ml milk

sunflower oil, for cooking

fruit, to serve (optional)

Directions

STEP 1

Heat the peanut butter, butter and 4 tbsp maple syrup in the microwave, or a pan, for 2 mins, stirring every 30 seconds until smooth and combined. Set aside to cool slightly.

STEP 2

Mix the flour, baking powder and sugar in a large bowl with a small pinch of salt. Crack in the eggs and whisk until smooth. Add the milk and ¾ of the peanut butter mixture and whisk to combine.

STEP 3

Heat a splash of sunflower oil and a small knob of butter in a non-stick frying pan until foaming. Add 2 tbsp of batter to make small pancakes, making sure there's space between each. Cook until bubbles start to form on the surface, then flip and cook on the other side. Keep warm in a low oven whilst you make the next batch.

STEP 4

Serve the pancakes with the remaining peanut butter sauce, maple syrup and fruit, if using. You may have to reheat the sauce to loosen the mixture slightly.

Spiced hot cross buns

Ingredients

For the dough

450g strong white flour, plus extra for dusting

2 x 7g sachets easy-blend yeast

50g caster sugar

150ml warm milk

1 egg, beaten

50g unsalted butter, melted, plus extra for greasing

oil, for greasing

The spices and dried fruit

1 tsp ground cinnamon

½ tsp mixed spice

¼ tsp grated nutmeg

100g currant

To decorate

4 tbsp plain flour

2 tbsp granulated sugar

Directions

STEP 1

Put the flour, yeast, caster sugar and 1 tsp salt into a large mixing bowl with the spices and dried fruit and mix well. Make a well in the centre and pour in the warm milk, 50ml warm water, the beaten egg and the melted butter. Mix everything together to form a dough – start with a wooden spoon and finish with your hands. If the dough is too dry, add a little more warm water; if it's too wet, add more flour.

STEP 2

Knead in the bowl or on a floured surface until the dough becomes smooth and springy. Transfer to a clean, lightly greased bowl and cover loosely with a clean, damp tea towel. Leave in a warm place to rise until roughly doubled in size – this will take about 1 hr depending on how warm the room is.

STEP 3

Tip the risen dough onto a lightly floured surface. Knead for a few secs, then divide into 12 even portions – I roll my dough into a long sausage shape, then quarter and divide each quarter into 3 pieces. Shape each portion into a smooth round and place on a baking sheet greased with butter, leaving some room between each bun for it to rise.

STEP 4

Use a small, sharp knife to score a cross on the top of each bun, then cover with the damp tea towel again and leave in a warm place to prove for 20 mins until almost doubled in size again. Heat oven to 200C/180C fan/gas 6.

STEP 5

When the buns are ready to bake, mix the plain flour with just enough water to give you a thick paste. Spoon into a piping bag (or into a plastic food bag and snip the corner off) and pipe a white cross into the crosses you cut earlier. Bake for 12-15 mins until the buns are golden and sound hollow when tapped on the bottom. While still warm, melt the granulated sugar with 1 tbsp water in a small pan, then brush over the buns.

Berry omelette

Ingredients

1 large egg

1 tbsp skimmed milk

3 pinches of cinnamon

½ tsp rapeseed oil

100g cottage cheese

175g chopped strawberry, blueberries and raspberries

Directions

STEP 1

Beat egg with milk and cinnamon. Heat oil in a 20cm non-stick frying pan and pour in the egg mixture, swirling to evenly cover the base. Cook for a few mins until set and golden underneath. There's no need to flip it over.

STEP 2

Place on a plate, spread over cheese, then scatter with berries. Roll up and serve.

Peanut butter & banana on toast

Ingredients

2 slices granary bread

1 small banana

½ tsp cinnamon

1 tbsp crunchy peanut butter

Directions

STEP 1

Toast bread and slice banana. Layer banana on one slice of toast and dust with cinnamon. Spread the second slice with peanut butter, then sandwich the two together and eat straight away.

Vegan breakfast muffins

Ingredients

150g muesli mix

50g light brown soft sugar

160g plain flour

1 tsp baking powder

250ml sweetened soy milk

1 apple, peeled and grated

2 tbsp grapeseed oil

3 tbsp nut butter (almond)

4 tbsp demerara sugar

50g pecans, roughly chilled

Directions

STEP 1

Heat the oven to 200C/180C fan/gas 6. Line a muffin tin with cases. Mix 100g muesli with the light brown sugar, flour and baking powder in a bowl. Combine the milk, apple, oil and 2 tbsp nut butter in a jug, then stir into the dry mixture. Divide equally between the cases. Mix the remaining muesli with the demerara sugar, remaining nut butter and the pecans, and spoon over the muffins.

STEP 2

Bake for 25-30 mins or until the muffins are risen and golden. Will keep for two to three days in an airtight container or freeze for one month. Refresh in the oven before serving.

Really easy cinnamon rolls

Ingredients

350g can ready-made croissant dough (we used Jus Rol)

30g unsalted butter, softened

2 tsp cinnamon

6 tbsp soft light brown sugar

Directions

STEP 1

Heat oven to 180C/160C fan/gas 4. Line a 23cm cake tin with a square of baking parchment so the corners stick up (this will help you to lift the rolls out).

STEP 2

Unroll the croissant dough from the can and lay it out on your work surface. Cut it into three sections along the dotted lines, but don't cut the diagonal line. Spread over a quarter of the butter onto each piece.

STEP 3

Mix the cinnamon and sugar together. Using one square of dough at a time, sprinkle over 2-3 tsp of the sugar and roll up the dough. When you have three rolls, cut each one in half and then each half into three. Arrange the rolls in the tin in two circles – you need to spread them well apart as they will rise and spread. Stick the end bits in among fatter pieces from the centre of the rolls so they cook evenly. Bake for 15 mins or until the rolls are risen and cooked through.

STEP 4

Meanwhile, heat the remaining sugar mix with the remaining butter until you have a thick caramel (don't worry if some of the butter separates out, it will soak into the dough). When the rolls are cooked, pour over the caramel. Leave to cool a little, then eat warm.

Bacon, brie and red onion baguettes

Ingredients

1 large white baguette, sliced into 4

8 rashers of smoked back bacon, grilled

200g brie, cut into slices (or chunks)

4 tbsp red onion chutney

Directions

STEP 1

Heat your oven to 200C/180C fan/gas 6. Slice the baguette sections vertically and fill each with 2 slices of bacon and a quarter of the cheese. Put them on a baking sheet. Cook in the oven for 5 mins, until the bread is crisped up and the cheese is beginning to melt.

STEP 2

Top each with a dollop of red onion chutney and serve immediately.

Healthy pesto eggs on toast

Ingredients

2-4 thin slices rye sourdough (about 70g total, depending on the size of the loaf)

2 eggs

170g tomatoes on-the-vine

160g baby spinach

pinch of chilli flakes (optional)

For the pesto

1 garlic clove

10g basil

1 tbsp pine nuts

1 tbsp rapeseed oil

1 tbsp finely grated parmesan or vegetarian alternative

Directions

STEP 1

To make the pesto, peel the garlic clove and put in a small food processor along with the basil, pine nuts, oil and 2 tbsp water. Blitz until smooth, then stir in the cheese. Or, blitz using a hand blender.

STEP 2

Toast the bread and divide between two plates. Cook the pesto in a frying pan over a medium heat for 30 seconds, stirring. Crack the eggs into one side of the pan, put the tomatoes in the other, and fry in the pesto until the eggs are cooked to your liking.

STEP 3

Lift out the eggs and put each one on a slice of toast. Add the spinach to the pan with the tomatoes, turn the heat up to high and cook until wilted, about 2-3 mins. The tomatoes should be soft. Spoon the veg onto the other toast slice and sprinkle with the chilli flakes, if you like.

Vegan bacon

Ingredients

250g vital wheat gluten, plus extra for dusting

50g gram (chickpea) flour

½ tsp garlic granules

½ tsp onion granules

½ tsp smoked paprika

25g nutritional yeast

1 tbsp maple syrup

30g tomato purée

2 tsp Dijon mustard

150ml vegetable stock

1 tsp liquid smoke flavouring

4 tbsp soy sauce

2 tbsp vegetable oil

For the glaze

60ml maple syrup

60ml soy sauce

1 tbsp tomato purée

½ tsp liquid smoke flavouring

½ tsp onion granules

½ tsp garlic granules

½ tsp smoked paprika

Directions

STEP 1

Heat the oven to 190C/170C fan/gas 5. Put the vital wheat gluten, gram flour, garlic and onion granules, paprika and nutritional yeast in a large bowl, and mix well with a wooden spoon. Stir the maple syrup, tomato purée, mustard, stock, liquid smoke and soy sauce together in a large jug.

STEP 2

Make a well in the dry Ingredients and pour in the wet, then stir together with a wooden spoon to combine. Tip out onto a lightly floured work surface and knead for 5 mins. Press into a 20cm non-stick round or square tin and bake for 20-30 mins until golden brown. Remove from the tin and leave to cool.

STEP 3

Put all the glaze Ingredients in a saucepan and stir to combine. Warm gently over a medium-low heat for 5 mins until the liquid is thick and glossy. Remove from the heat and set aside. Slice the cooled 'bacon' into 3mm-thick slices.

STEP 4

Heat about 4 tsp of the oil in a large, non-stick pan over a medium heat. Meanwhile, brush each side of the 'bacon' rashers with the glaze and fry, in batches, for 1-2 mins on each side until dark brown.

Transfer to a plate and let stand for a few minutes to crisp up. Serve warm.

DELICIOUS INTERSTITIAL CYSTITIS DIET LUNCH RECIPES

Roast mushroom gnocchi

Ingredients

250g mushrooms

500g fresh gnocchi

3 tbsp olive oil, plus extra for drizzling

160g bag spinach

100g blue cheese

Directions

STEP 1

Heat oven to 220C/200C fan/gas 7. Slice the mushrooms and put in a roasting tin with the gnocchi, then drizzle over 3 tbsp olive oil. Roast for 25-30 mins or until the gnocchi are golden, stirring occasionally to stop them sticking.

STEP 2

Once the gnocchi are ready, stir half the spinach into the tin to wilt it, then crumble the blue cheese over the top. Put it back in the oven just to melt the cheese, then serve with the remaining spinach, drizzled with a little olive oil.

Vegan curried squash, lentil & coconut soup

Ingredients

1 tbsp olive oil

1 butternut squash, peeled, deseeded and diced

200g carrot, diced

1 tbsp curry powder containing turmeric

100g red lentil

700ml low-sodium vegetable stock

1 can reduced-fat coconut milk

coriander and naan bread, to serve

Directions

STEP 1

Heat the oil in a large saucepan, add the squash and carrots, sizzle for 1 min, then stir in the curry powder and cook for 1 min more. Tip in the lentils, the vegetable stock and coconut milk and give everything a good stir. Bring to the boil, then turn the heat down and simmer for 15-18 mins until everything is tender.

STEP 2

Using a hand blender or in a food processor, blitz until as smooth as you like. Season and serve scattered with roughly chopped coriander and some naan bread alongside.

Salade niçoise

Ingredients

8 new potatoes

50g green beans (or a small handful), trimmed and halved

3 eggs

2 Little Gem lettuces, quartered

50g pitted black olives

2 medium tomatoes (plum are good), quartered

145g can tuna in olive oil, drained, oil reserved (see below)

For the dressing

½ garlic clove

1 anchovy fillet (optional)

1 tbsp Dijion mustard

2 tbsp red wine vinegar

4 tbsp reserved olive oil from the tuna can (topped up, if needed)

Directions

STEP 1

To make the dressing, mash the garlic and anchovy, if using, with a small pinch of salt on a board using the blade of a large knife, or in a pestle and mortar.

Combine the paste with the mustard and vinegar, then slowly stir in the tuna oil. Set aside.

STEP 2

Tip the new potatoes into a large pan of cold salted water, ensuring they're well covered. Bring to the boil, then reduce the heat to a simmer. Add the beans and cook for 5 mins, then remove with a slotted spoon and immediately plunge into a bowl of iced water to cool. Cook the potatoes for another 5 mins until tender, then drain and leave to cool. When cool enough to handle, halve or quarter them, and toss in a large bowl with 1 tbsp of the dressing. Leave to cool completely.

STEP 3

Meanwhile, cook the eggs in a second pan of simmering water for 7½ mins, then transfer to a bowl of iced water to cool. Drain the beans and eggs, then peel and halve the eggs.

STEP 4

Tip the lettuce quarters, cooked beans and olives into the bowl with the potatoes. Add most of the remaining dressing and gently toss. Divide the salad between two bowls, and top with the tomatoes and eggs. Flake over the tuna, then drizzle with the rest of the dressing and season.

Pan-fried chicken in mushroom sauce

Ingredients

2 tbsp sunflower oil

6 large, free-range chicken legs, halved at the joint
so you have 6 thighs and 6 drumsticks

700ml/1¼ pts chicken stock (or water)

50g butter

1 onion, finely diced

400g mixed wild mushrooms

300ml/½ pt dry white wine

284ml pot double cream

Directions

STEP 1

Heat the oil in a large non-stick frying pan. Fry the thighs for 8-10 mins, skin side only, until golden brown, then transfer to a casserole dish. Fry the drumsticks for about 5 mins each side and add them to the thighs.

STEP 2

Pour the stock over the chicken legs in the casserole. There should be enough stock to just cover the chicken, if not add a little water. Bring stock to the boil and cover, leaving lid slightly ajar.

Cook at just below simmering point for 30-35 mins until chicken is cooked.

STEP 3

While chicken is simmering, drain oil from the pan. Heat the butter in pan and add onion. Sweat onion for 5 mins until soft, but not coloured. Turn up the heat, add the mushrooms, then fry for 3 mins until they soften and start to smell wonderful. Pour over the white wine, raise the heat to maximum and boil rapidly for 6-8 mins until reduced by two-thirds. Turn off the heat and leave until chicken has cooked.

STEP 4

Once chicken legs are cooked, strain stock into pan with the onion, mushrooms and white wine, bring back to the boil and reduce again by two-thirds until it is thick and syrupy. Pour in double cream, bring it to the boil, season if you want, then pour it over chicken. Heat chicken through in the sauce for 2-3 mins then turn off the heat and leave for a few mins before serving. This is such an aromatic and beautiful looking dish you should serve it straight from the casserole with the lid on.

Easy salmon sushi rice bowl

Ingredients

150g sushi rice

pinch of caster sugar

1 tbsp rice vinegar

120g frozen edamame

1 large carrot

handful of radishes

¼ cucumber

2 cooked skinless salmon fillets

1-2 tbsp soy sauce

1 tsp toasted sesame seeds

few pieces of sushi ginger, optional

Equipment

scales

measuring jug

medium saucepan with a lid

measuring spoons

wooden spoon

small saucepan

vegetable peeler

chopping board

sharp knife

Directions

STEP 1

Tip the sushi rice into a medium saucepan, cover with 200ml water and add a pinch of salt. Put the pan on the hob and turn the heat to high. Wait for the water to boil, then reduce the heat to very low, cover the pan with a lid and leave to gently cook for 15 mins.

STEP 2

After 15 mins turn off the heat, fluff up the rice with a fork, then return the lid to the pan and leave for another 5 mins, the rice will continue to cook. After

5 mins, check the rice is cooked – it should have absorbed all the water and be soft but not mushy. Stir the sugar and vinegar through the rice, cover with the lid again and leave to keep warm while you prepare the other Ingredients.

STEP 3

Fill a small pan halfway with water, put it on the hob and bring the water to a gentle boil. Add the edamame beans, cook for 3 mins, then carefully drain.

STEP 4

Peel the carrot and discard the outer skin, then keep peeling the flesh to create lots of carrot ribbons.

STEP 5

Thinly slice the radishes. Cut the cucumber into batons, then thinly slice lengthways.

STEP 6

With your hands, break the salmon into small pieces – look out for any bones and throw these away.

STEP 7

Divide the warm rice between two bowls and arrange the other Ingredients on top, then drizzle with the soy sauce and sesame seeds, and add a few pieces of sushi ginger, if using.

Prawn & salmon burgers with spicy mayo

Ingredients

180g pack peeled raw prawns, roughly chopped

4 skinless salmon fillets, chopped into small chunks

3 spring onions, roughly chopped

1 lemon, zested and juiced

small pack coriander

60g mayonnaise or Greek yogurt

4 tsp chilli sauce (we used sriracha)

2 Little Gem lettuces, shredded

1 cucumber, peeled into ribbons

1 tbsp olive oil

4 seeded burger buns, toasted, to serve

Directions

STEP 1

Briefly blitz half the prawns, half the salmon, the spring onions, lemon zest and half the coriander in a food processor until it forms a coarse paste. Tip into a bowl, stir in the rest of the prawns and salmon, season well and shape into four burgers. Chill for 10 mins.

STEP 2

Mix the mayo and chilli sauce together in a small bowl, season and add some lemon juice to taste. Mix the lettuce with the cucumber, dress with a little of the remaining lemon juice and 1 tsp olive oil, then set aside.

STEP 3

Heat the remaining oil in a large frying pan and fry the burgers for 3-4 mins each side or until they have a nice crust and the fish is cooked through. Serve with the salad on the side or in toasted burger buns, if you like, with a good dollop of the spicy mayo.

Roast chicken traybake

Ingredients

2 red onions (320g), sliced across into rings

1 large red pepper, deseeded and chopped into 3cm pieces

300g potatoes, peeled and cut into 3cm chunks

2 tbsp rapeseed oil

4 bone-in chicken thighs, skin and any fat removed

1 lime, zested and juiced

3 large garlic cloves, finely grated

1 tsp smoked paprika

1 tsp thyme leaves

2 tsp vegetable bouillon powder

200g long stem broccoli, stem cut into lengths if very thick

Directions

STEP 1

Heat the oven to 200C/180C fan/gas 6. Put the onion, pepper, potatoes and oil in a non-stick roasting tin and toss everything together. Roast for 15 mins while you rub the chicken with the lime zest, garlic, paprika and thyme. Take the veg from the oven, stir, then snuggle the chicken thighs among the veg, covering them with some of the onions so they don't dry out as it roasts for 40 mins.

STEP 2

As you approach the end of the cooking time, mix
200ml boiling water with the bouillon powder. Take
the roasting tin from the oven, add the broccoli to
the tin, and pour over the hot stock followed by the
lime juice, then quickly cover with the foil and put
back in the oven for 10 more mins until the broccoli
is just tender.

Mushroom & spinach risotto

Ingredients

1 tbsp olive oil

25g butter

1 onion, chopped

140g chestnut mushrooms, sliced

1 fat garlic clove, crushed

140g arborio rice

150ml dry white wine

4 sundried tomatoes, chopped

500ml hot vegetable stock

2 tbsp chopped fresh parsley

25g parmesan or vegetarian alternative, freshly grated

100g fresh young leaf spinach, washed if necessary

warm ciabatta and green salad, to serve

Directions

STEP 1

Heat the oil and butter in a large deep frying pan. Add the onion and cook gently for 5 minutes until softened. Stir in the mushrooms and garlic and cook gently for 2-3 minutes.

STEP 2

Stir in the rice to coat with the onion and mushroom mixture. Pour in the wine and cook over a moderate heat for about 3 minutes, stirring from time to time, until the wine is absorbed.

STEP 3

Reduce to a gentle heat. Add the tomatoes and 125ml/ 4fl oz of the stock and cook for about 5 minutes until the liquid is absorbed. Pour in a further 125ml/4fl oz stock and continue cooking until absorbed. Repeat with the remaining stock, until it is all absorbed and the rice is creamy and tender.

STEP 4

Stir in the parsley and half the parmesan. Season to taste. Scatter the spinach over the risotto. Cover and cook gently for 4-5 minutes until the spinach has just wilted. Serve immediately sprinkled with the remaining parmesan.

Mustardy salmon with beetroot & lentils

Ingredients

2 tbsp olive oil

1 tbsp wholegrain mustard

½ tsp honey

2 salmon fillets

250g pouch ready-cooked puy lentils

250g pack ready-cooked beetroot, cut into wedges

2 tbsp crème fraîche

1 small pack dill, roughly chopped

1-2 tbsp capers

½ lemon, zested and cut into 2 wedges to serve

2 tbsp pumpkin seeds, toasted

rocket, to serve (optional)

Directions

STEP 1

Heat oven to 200C/180C fan/gas 6. Mix together 1 tbsp oil, the mustard, honey and some seasoning. Put the salmon fillets on a baking tray and spread the honey and mustard mixture all over. Tip the lentils and beetroot into a casserole dish, toss with the remaining oil and season well. Put both in the oven for 10 mins until the salmon is cooked through.

STEP 2

Stir the crème fraîche, dill, capers and lemon zest through the lentils. Serve alongside the salmon with the pumpkin seeds scattered over and lemon wedges for squeezing, with a rocket salad on the side, if you like.

Curried kale & chickpea soup

Ingredients

1 tsp rapeseed or coconut oil

1 onion, chopped

1 tbsp grated ginger

2 garlic cloves, crushed

1 sweet potato (about 200g), peeled and cut into 2cm cubes

1 tsp turmeric

2 tsp ground cumin

2 tbsp medium or hot curry powder

400g can chickpeas, rinsed

150ml low-fat coconut milk

500ml vegetable stock (see tip, below)

160g kale, chopped

1 lime, juiced

1 red chilli, finely chopped (optional)

Directions

STEP 1

Heat the oil in a large pan and fry the onion for 5 mins. Add the ginger and garlic, fry for 1 min more, then stir in the sweet potato, spices and chickpeas. Cook for another 5 mins, adding a little water if the spices stick to the pan.

STEP 2

Pour in the coconut milk and 400ml of the stock, then bring to a simmer and cook for 8 mins. Season, then transfer a quarter of the soup to a blender and whizz until smooth. Pour in the reserved stock to loosen, if needed, then add back to the pan with the remaining soup. Stir in the kale and cook for 5 mins. Add the lime juice, then ladle into bowls and scatter over the chilli, if you like.

Crab & asparagus pappardelle

Ingredients

1 tbsp olive oil

pinch of fennel seeds

½ red chilli, finely chopped

2 shallots, finely chopped

small bunch parsley, stalks finely chopped, leaves roughly chopped

½ lemon, zested and juiced

1 tbsp tomato purée

50ml vermouth

1 dressed crab (about 120g white and brown meat)

200g fresh egg pappardelle

200g asparagus, woody stalks removed, sliced on the diagonal (fatter stalks sliced in half lengthways)

1 tbsp crème fraîche

1 tbsp snipped chives

handful chopped hazelnuts

Directions

STEP 1

Heat the olive oil in a heavy-bottomed frying pan. Add the fennel seeds, chilli, shallots, parsley stalks, lemon zest and seasoning, and fry for about 5 mins, or until softened and aromatic. Add the tomato purée, cook for a couple of mins, then deglaze with the vermouth. Add half the crabmeat, stir to create a thick sauce, then remove from the heat while you cook the pasta.

STEP 2

Bring a large pan of salted water to the boil and cook the pasta until al dente. With 3 mins remaining, add the asparagus, then use a slotted spoon to transfer the pasta and asparagus to the crab pan. Put the crab pan back on the heat, add a couple of spoonfuls of pasta water to loosen and toss together, coating the pasta in the sauce. Add the rest of the crabmeat, crème fraîche and lemon juice, and warm through. Divide between plates and garnish with parsley, chives and hazelnuts.

Air-fryer cheese & ham toastie

Ingredients

20g butter, softened

2 slices sourdough or other bread

½ tsp English mustard

50g grated mature cheddar or gruyère

1 tbsp chopped chives (optional)

1 thick slice of ham

Directions

STEP 1

Heat the air-fryer to 190C. Butter the slices of bread on one side each, then combine the remaining butter with the mustard, cheese and chives, if using. Season with black pepper.

STEP 2

Spread the cheese mixture over the plain sides of the bread, then sandwich the ham between the two slices so the buttered sides are facing out. Air-fry for 10 mins, turning once until golden and crunchy on the outside, and the cheese has melted in the middle.

Leek, cheese & bacon tart

Ingredients

1 tbsp olive oil

3 leeks, thinly sliced

375g pack ready-rolled puff pastry

150g pack soft cheese with garlic and herbs

4 rashers streaky bacon, snipped

100g grated emmental

Directions

STEP 1

Heat oven to 200C/180C fan/gas 6. Heat the oil in a frying pan, then gently fry the leeks until soft, about 5 mins. Cool. Unroll the pastry onto a baking sheet. Spread the soft cheese over the pastry to within 3cm of the edges. Scatter over the leeks, bacon and grated emmental.

STEP 2

Flip the edges of the pastry over the filling. Bake for 20 mins until golden.

Microwave sweet & sour chicken

Ingredients

9 tbsp tomato ketchup

3 tbsp malt vinegar

4 tbsp dark muscovado sugar

2 garlic cloves, crushed

4 skinless and boneless chicken breast, cut into chunks

1 small onion, roughly chopped

2 red peppers, seeded and cut into chunks

227g can pineapple pieces in juice, drained

100g sugar snap peas, roughly sliced

handful salted, roasted cashew nuts, optional

Directions

STEP 1

In a large microwaveable dish, mix the ketchup, vinegar, sugar and garlic thoroughly with the chicken, onion and peppers. Microwave, uncovered, on high for 8-10 mins until the chicken is starting to cook and the sauce is sizzling.

STEP 2

Stir in the pineapple pieces and sugar snap peas and return to the microwave for another 3-5 mins until the chicken is completely cooked. Leave to stand for a few minutes, then stir in the cashews, if using, and

serve.

DELICIOUS INTERSTITIAL CYSTITIS DIET DINNER RECIPES

Pasta primavera

Ingredients

75g young broad beans (use frozen if you can't get fresh)

2 x 100g pack asparagus tips

170g peas (use frozen if you can't get fresh)

350g spaghetti or tagliatelle

175g pack baby leeks, trimmed and sliced

1 tbsp olive oil, plus extra to serve

1 tbsp butter

200ml tub fromage frais or creme fraiche

handful fresh chopped herbs (we used mint, parsley and chives)

parmesan (or vegetarian alternative), shaved, to serve

Direction

STEP 1

Bring a pan of salted water to the boil and put a steamer (or colander) over the water. Steam the beans, asparagus and peas until just tender, then set aside. Boil the pasta following pack instructions.

STEP 2

Meanwhile, fry the leeks gently in the oil and butter for 5 mins or until soft. Add the fromage frais to the leeks and very gently warm through, stirring constantly to ensure it doesn't split. Add the herbs and steamed vegetables with a splash of pasta water to loosen.

STEP 3

Drain the pasta and stir into the sauce. Adjust the seasoning, then serve scattered with the cheese and drizzled with a little extra olive oil.

Pork & chilli lettuce cups

Ingredients

1 tbsp vegetable oil

1 shallot, thinly sliced

1 lemongrass stalk, finely chopped

4 garlic cloves, grated

1 birds-eye chilli, finely chopped

500g pork mince

1 tbsp fish sauce

1 tsp dark brown soft sugar

2 limes, juiced

2 Little Gem lettuces, leaves separated

thinly sliced spring onions, shredded carrots, finely chopped coriander leaves and mint leaves, to serve

Direction

STEP 1

Heat the oil in a large frying pan over a medium heat and fry the shallot, lemongrass, garlic and chilli for 3 mins until fragrant. Add the pork mince and stir-fry for about 10 mins more until the pork is cooked through and browned. Add the fish sauce, sugar and lime juice, and cook for a couple more minutes until the pork is coated in the mixture. To freeze, leave to cool completely, then transfer to a freezer bag, seal and lay flat in the freezer (so the mince stays in a thin layer). Will keep for up to two months. Defrost in the fridge overnight before using. Reheat in a dry frying pan over a low heat until piping hot.

STEP 2

Divide the pork mince between the lettuce leaves and garnish with the spring onions, carrots and herbs, then serve.

Jerk sweet potato & black bean curry

Ingredients

2 onions, 1 diced, 1 roughly chopped

2 tbsp sunflower oil

50g ginger, roughly chopped

small bunch coriander, leaves and stalks separated

3 tbsp jerk seasoning

2 thyme sprigs

400g can chopped tomato

4 tbsp red wine vinegar

3 tbsp demerara sugar

2 vegetable stock cubes, crumbled

1kg sweet potato, peeled and cut into chunks

2 x 400g cans black beans, rinsed and drained

450g jar roasted red pepper, cut into thick slices

Direction

STEP 1

Gently soften the diced onion in the sunflower oil in a big pan or casserole.

STEP 2

Meanwhile, whizz together the roughly chopped onion, ginger, coriander stalks and jerk seasoning with a hand-held blender. Add to the softened onion and fry until fragrant. Stir in the thyme, chopped tomatoes, vinegar, sugar and stock cubes with 600ml water and bring to a simmer. Simmer for 10 mins, then drop in the sweet potatoes and simmer for 10 mins more. Stir in the beans, peppers and some seasoning, and simmer for another 5 mins until the potatoes are almost tender. Cool and chill for up to 2 days.

STEP 3

To serve, gently heat through on the hob. Roughly chop most of the coriander leaves and stir in, then serve scattered with the remaining leaves.

Chicken tacos

Ingredients

250g plain flour, plus extra for dusting

2 tbsp rapeseed oil

2 tbsp taco or fajita seasoning (see tip, below)

5-6 skinless chicken breasts, sliced

¼ red cabbage, finely shredded

3 limes, 1 juiced, 2 cut into wedges

small bunch of coriander, chopped

4 sweetcorn cob, kernels sliced off, or 400g frozen sweetcorn

400g can black beans, drained and rinsed

2 garlic cloves, crushed

4 tbsp fat-free yogurt, to serve

chilli sauce, to serve

Direction

STEP 1

Combine the flour with half the oil and a small pinch of salt in a bowl. Pour over 125-150ml warm water, then bring together into a soft dough with your hands. Cut into six equal pieces, then cut four of the pieces in half again, so you have eight small pieces and two large. Roll all the pieces out on a floured work surface until they're as thin as you can get them.

STEP 2

Heat a dry frying pan over a medium-high heat and cook the small and large tortillas for 2-3 mins on each side until golden and toasted (do this one at a time). Leave the large tortillas to cool, then cover and reserve for use in the lunchboxes (see tip below). Keep the small tortillas warm in foil.

STEP 3

Sprinkle the taco seasoning over the chicken in a bowl, and toss to combine. Toss the cabbage with the lime juice, half the coriander and some seasoning in another bowl, then leave to pickle.

STEP 4

Meanwhile, heat two frying pans over a high heat. Divide the remaining oil between the pans and fry the sweetcorn and a pinch of salt until sizzling and turning golden, stirring occasionally – you want the sweetcorn to char slightly, as this adds flavour, so you may need to leave it to cook undisturbed for a bit. While the sweetcorn cooks and chars, fry the chicken in the larger pan until cooked through and golden (you may need to do this in batches).

STEP 5

Tip the black beans and garlic into the sweetcorn and stir to warm through. Squeeze over two of the lime wedges.

STEP 6

Reserve two spoonfuls each of the chicken (about 1 chicken breast) and sweetcorn mix for use in the lunchboxes (see tip, below), then serve the rest in bowls alongside the cabbage, yogurt, lime wedges, remaining coriander, chilli sauce and tortillas for everyone to dig into

Mediterranean fish stew with garlic toasts

Ingredients

3 tbsp olive oil

1 large onion, sliced

2 garlic cloves, sliced

1 red chilli, finely chopped

2 tbsp tomato purée

1kg tomatoes, roughly chopped

200ml white wine

350ml fish stock

3 strips orange zest

1kg skinless halibut fillets, cut into large chunks

500g clams

400g large raw prawns

handful flat-leaf parsley, chopped

For the garlic toasts

1 large ciabatta loaf, cut into 1cm slices

5 tbsp olive oil

2 garlic cloves, halved

Direction

STEP 1

To make the garlic toasts, drizzle the bread with oil, then griddle or grill until golden all over. While the toasts are still hot, rub them with garlic and set aside.

STEP 2

Heat the oil in a wide, deep frying pan. Add the onion and cook over a gentle heat for 5 mins until softened. Stir through the garlic and chilli and cook a couple of mins more. Add the tomato purée and tomatoes. Turn up the heat and cook for 10-15 mins, stirring until the tomatoes are pulpy. Pour over the wine and cook for 10 mins more until most of it has boiled away.

STEP 3

Add the fish stock and orange zest and heat until gently simmering. Nestle the halibut chunks into the liquid and cook for 5 mins. Add the clams and prawns and cook for 5 mins more until the fish is cooked through and the clams have opened (discard any that haven't). Sprinkle the parsley over the stew and serve with the garlic toasts.

Chicken with crushed harissa chickpeas

Ingredients

2 tbsp rapeseed oil

1 onion, chopped

1 red pepper, finely sliced

1 yellow pepper, finely sliced

4 chicken breasts

1 tbsp za'atar

400g can chickpeas

1½ tbsp red harissa paste

150g baby spinach

½ small bunch of parsley, finely chopped

lemon wedges, to serve

Direction

STEP 1

Heat 1 tbsp of oil in a frying pan over a medium heat and fry the onions and peppers for 7 mins until softened and golden.

STEP 2

Meanwhile, put the chicken between two sheets of baking parchment and lightly bash until about 2cm thick. Mix together the remaining oil and the za'atar, then rub over the chicken. Season to taste.

STEP 3

Heat the grill to high. Put the chicken on a baking tray lined with foil, and grill for 3-4 mins each side, or until golden and cooked through.

STEP 4

Heat the chickpeas in a pan with the harissa paste and 2 tbsp water until warmed through, then roughly mash with a potato masher. Wilt the spinach in a pan with 1 tbsp of water or in the microwave in a heatproof bowl. Stir the pepper and onion mixture, spinach and parsley through the chickpeas. Serve with the sliced chicken and the lemon wedges for squeezing over.

Healthy egg & chips

Ingredients

500g potatoes, diced

2 shallots, sliced

1 tbsp olive oil

2 tsp dried crushed oregano or 1 tsp fresh leaves

200g small mushroom

4 eggs

Direction

STEP 1

Heat oven to 200C/fan 180C/gas 6. Tip the potatoes and shallots into a large, non-stick roasting tin, drizzle with the oil, sprinkle over the oregano, then mix everything together well. Bake for 40-45 mins (or until starting to go brown), add the mushrooms, then cook for a further 10 mins until the potatoes are browned and tender.

STEP 2

Make four gaps in the vegetables and crack an egg into each space. Return to the oven for 3-4 mins or until the eggs are cooked to your liking.

Pot-roast beef with French onion gravy

Ingredients

1kg silverside or topside of beef with no added fat

2 tbsp olive oil

8 young carrots, tops trimmed (but leave a little, if you like)

1 celery stick, finely chopped

200ml white wine

600ml rich beef stock

2 bay leaves

500g onion

a few thyme sprigs

1 tsp butter

1 tsp light brown or light muscovado sugar

2 tsp plain flour

Direction

STEP 1

Heat oven to 160C/140C fan/gas 3. Rub the meat with 1 tsp of the oil and plenty of seasoning. Heat a large flameproof casserole dish and brown the meat all over for about 10 mins. Meanwhile, add 2 tsp oil to a frying pan and fry the carrots and celery for 10 mins until turning golden.

STEP 2

Lift the beef onto a plate, splash the wine into the hot casserole and boil for 2 mins. Pour in the stock, return the beef, then tuck in the carrots, celery and bay leaves, trying not to submerge the carrots too much. Cover and cook in the oven for 2 hrs. (I like to turn the beef halfway through cooking.)

STEP 3

Meanwhile, thinly slice the onions. Heat 1 tbsp oil in a pan and stir in the onions, thyme and some seasoning. Cover and cook gently for 20 mins until the onions are softened but not coloured. Remove the lid, turn up the heat, add the butter and sugar, then let the onions caramelise to a dark golden brown, stirring often. Remove the thyme sprigs, then set aside.

STEP 4

When the beef is ready, it will be tender and easy to pull apart at the edges. Remove it from the casserole and snip off the strings. Reheat the onion pan, stir in the flour and cook for 1 min. Whisk the floury onions into the beefy juices in the casserole, to make a thick onion gravy. Taste for seasoning. Add the beef and carrots back to the casserole, or slice the beef and bring to the table on a platter, with the carrots to the side and the gravy spooned over.

Vegan chickpea curry jacket potatoes

Ingredients

4 sweet potatoes

1 tbsp coconut oil

1 ½ tsp cumin seeds

1 large onion, diced

2 garlic cloves, crushed

thumb-sized piece ginger, finely grated

1 green chilli, finely chopped

1 tsp garam masala

1 tsp ground coriander

½ tsp turmeric

2 tbsp tikka masala paste

2 x 400g can chopped tomatoes

2 x 400g can chickpeas, drained

lemon wedges and coriander leaves, to serve

Direction

STEP 1

Heat oven to 200C/180C fan/gas 6. Prick the sweet potatoes all over with a fork, then put on a baking tray and roast in the oven for 45 mins or until tender when pierced with a knife.

STEP 2

Meanwhile, melt the coconut oil in a large saucepan over medium heat. Add the cumin seeds and fry for 1 min until fragrant, then add the onion and fry for 7-10 mins until softened.

STEP 3

Put the garlic, ginger and green chilli into the pan, and cook for 2-3 mins. Add the spices and tikka masala paste and cook for a further 2 mins until fragrant, then tip in the tomatoes. Bring to a simmer, then tip in the chickpeas and cook for a further 20 mins until thickened. Season.

STEP 4

Put the roasted sweet potatoes on four plates and cut open lengthways. Spoon over the chickpea curry and squeeze over the lemon wedges. Season, then scatter with coriander before serving.

Chipotle chicken

Ingredients

1 onion, chopped

1 garlic clove, sliced

2 tbsp sunflower oil

1-2 tbsp chipotle paste (see tip, below)

400g can chopped tomatoes

1 tbsp cider vinegar

8 skinless chicken thigh fillets

small bunch coriander, chopped

soured cream and rice, to serve

Direction

STEP 1

Fry the onion and garlic in the oil in a deep, wide frying pan until soft. Add the chipotle paste (use 1 tbsp for a mild flavour and 2 tbsp for a hotter, stronger one). Stir and cook for 1 min, then add the tomatoes and cider vinegar. Bring to a simmer and cook for 10 mins with the lid half on. Stir to make sure it doesn't get too dry.

STEP 2

Add the chicken and cook for 10 mins or until cooked through, turning once. Scatter with coriander and serve with rice and soured cream.

Winter vegetable & lentil soup

Ingredients

85g dried red lentils

2 carrots, quartered lengthways then diced

3 sticks celery, sliced

2 small leeks, sliced

2 tbsp tomato purée

1 tbsp fresh thyme leaves

3 large garlic cloves, chopped

1 tbsp vegetable bouillon powder

1 heaped tsp ground coriander

Direction

STEP 1

Tip all the Ingredients into a large pan. Pour over
1½ litres boiling water, then stir well.

STEP 2

Cover and leave to simmer for 30 mins until the
vegetables and lentils are tender.

STEP 3

Ladle into bowls and eat straightaway, or if you like
a really thick texture, blitz a third of the soup with
a hand blender or in a food processor.

Spaghetti with sardines

Ingredients

400g spaghetti

1 tbsp olive oil

2 garlic cloves, crushed

pinch chilli flakes

227g can chopped tomato

2 cans skinless and boneless sardines in tomato sauce

100g pitted black olives, roughly chopped

1 tbsp capers, drained

small handful parsley, chopped

Direction

STEP 1

Cook the spaghetti in a large pan of boiling salted water according to pack instructions. Meanwhile, make the sauce. Heat the oil in a medium pan and cook the garlic for 1 min. Add the chilli flakes, tomatoes and sardines, breaking up roughly with a wooden spoon. Heat for 2-3 mins, then stir in the olives, capers and most of the parsley. Mix well to combine.

STEP 2

Drain the pasta, reserving a couple of tbsp of the water. Add the pasta to the sauce and mix well, adding the reserved water if the sauce is a little thick. Divide between 4 bowls and sprinkle with the remaining parsley.

Tuna, asparagus & white bean salad

Ingredients

1 large bunch asparagus

2 x cans tuna steaks in water, drained

2 x cans cannellini beans in water, drained

1 red onion, very finely chopped

2 tbsp capers

1 tbsp olive oil

1 tbsp red wine vinegar

2 tbsp tarragon, finely chopped

Direction

STEP 1

Cook the asparagus in a large pan of boiling water
for 4-5 mins until tender. Drain well, cool under
running water, then cut into finger-length pieces.
Toss together the tuna, beans, onion, capers and
asparagus in a large serving bowl.

STEP 2

Mix the oil, vinegar and tarragon together, then pour over the salad. Chill until ready to serve.

The ultimate makeover: Chicken pie

Ingredients

For the filling

450ml chicken stock, from a cube (I use Kallo, organic)

100ml white wine

2 garlic cloves, finely chopped

3 thyme sprigs

1 tarragon sprig, plus 1 tbsp chopped tarragon leaves

225g carrots, cut into batons

4 skinless chicken breasts, 500g/1lb 2oz total weight

225g leeks, sliced

2 tbsp cornflour, mixed with 2 tbsp water

3 tbsp crème fraîche

1 heaped tsp Dijon mustard

1 heaped tbsp chopped flat-leaf or curly parsley

For the topping

70g filo pastry (I used three 39 x 30cm sheets)

1 tbsp rapeseed oil

Direction

STEP 1

Pour the stock and wine into a large, wide frying pan. Add the garlic, thyme, tarragon sprig and carrots, bring to the boil then lower the heat and simmer for 3 mins. Lay the chicken in the stock, grind over some pepper, cover and simmer for 5 mins. Scatter the leek slices over the chicken, cover again then gently simmer for 10 more mins, so the leeks can steam while the chicken cooks. Remove from the heat and let the chicken sit in the stock for about 15 mins, so it keeps moist while cooling slightly.

STEP 2

Strain the stock into a jug – you should have 500ml (if not, make up with water). Tip the chicken and veg into a 1.5 litre pie dish and discard the herb sprigs. Pour the stock back into the sauté pan, then slowly pour in the cornflour mix. Return the pan to the heat and bring to the boil, stirring constantly, until thickened. Remove from the heat and stir in the crème fraîche, mustard, chopped tarragon and parsley. Season with pepper. Heat oven to 200C/180C fan/gas 6.

STEP 3

Tear or cut the chicken into chunky shreds. Pour the sauce over the chicken mixture, then stir everything together.

STEP 4

Cut each sheet of filo into 4 squares or rectangles. Layer them on top of the filling, brushing each sheet with some of the oil as you go. Lightly scrunch up the filo so it doesn't lie completely flat and tuck the edges into the sides of the dish, or lay them on the edges if the dish has a rim. Grind over a little pepper, place the dish on a baking sheet, then bake for 20-25 mins until the pastry is golden and the sauce is bubbling. Serve immediately.

DELICIOUS INTERSTITIAL CYSTITIS DIET SNACK RECIPES

Classic scones with jam & clotted cream

Ingredients

350g self-raising flour, plus more for dusting

1 tsp baking powder

85g butter, cut into cubes

3 tbsp caster sugar

175ml milk

1 tsp vanilla extract

squeeze lemon juice (see tips below)

beaten egg, to glaze

jam and clotted cream, to serve

Directions

STEP 1

Heat the oven to 220C/200C fan/gas 7. Tip the self-raising flour into a large bowl with ¼ tsp salt and the baking powder, then mix.

STEP 2

Add the butter, then rub in with your fingers until the mix looks like fine crumbs. Stir in the caster sugar.

STEP 3

Put the milk into a jug and heat in the microwave for about 30 secs until warm, but not hot. Add the vanilla extract and a squeeze of lemon juice, then set aside for a moment.

STEP 4

Put a baking tray in the oven. Make a well in the dry mix, then add the liquid and combine it quickly with a cutlery knife – it will seem pretty wet at first.

STEP 5

Scatter some flour onto the work surface and tip the dough out. Dredge the dough and your hands with a little more flour, then fold the dough over 2-3 times until it's a little smoother. Pat into a roundabout 4cm deep. Take a 5cm cutter (smooth-edged cutters tend to cut more cleanly, giving a better rise) and dip it into some flour. Plunge into the dough, then repeat until you have four scones. You may need to press what's left of the dough back into a round to cut out another four.

STEP 6

Brush the tops with a beaten egg, then carefully arrange on the hot baking tray. Bake for 10 mins until risen and golden on the top. Eat just warm or cold on the day of baking, generously topped with jam and clotted cream. If freezing, freeze once cool. Defrost, then put in a low oven (about 160C/140C fan/gas 3) for a few minutes to refresh.

Pea & bacon pasties

Ingredients

200g pack smoked bacon lardon, cut into small pieces

225g frozen pea

140g mascarpone

25g parmesan, grated, plus a little extra for the tops

2 medium eggs

small handful mint, leaves chopped

375g pack puff pastry

plain flour, for rolling

Directions

STEP 1

Put the lardons in a large frying pan, cook until crisp, about 8 mins, then drain on kitchen paper. Meanwhile, pour kettle-hot water over the peas and leave to stand for 5 mins, then drain well.

STEP 2

Heat oven to 200C/180C fan/gas 6. When the bacon and peas have cooled, combine in a large bowl. Mash lightly to crush the peas and break up the bacon. Stir in the mascarpone, Parmesan, 1 egg and the mint, then season with black pepper.

STEP 3

Roll out the pastry on a lightly floured surface to the thickness of a 20p coin. Cut circles out using an 12cm cutter. Spoon the filling into the centre of each. Brush the edges with beaten egg and pinch the pastry together on one side to seal. Brush the tops with a little more egg wash and sprinkle each with Parmesan. Place the pasties on 2 floured baking sheets. Bake for 25 mins. Leave to cool, then chill until ready to serve or pack up.

BLT pasta salad

Ingredients

25g pasta bows

2 cooked crispy bacon rashers, broken into pieces

15g spinach, chopped

6 cherry tomatoes, halved

½ tbsp crème fraîche

¼ tsp wholegrain mustard

Directions

STEP 1

The night before, cook the pasta following pack instructions and run under cold water to cool quickly. Mix in the bacon, spinach, tomatoes, crème fraîche and mustard, and season with a little salt. Spoon into an airtight container and keep overnight in the fridge.

Apple flapjacks

Ingredients

175g butter, plus extra for the tin

2-3 apples (about 350g), peeled, cored and chopped into small pieces

200g golden syrup

150g light brown soft sugar

300g porridge oats

50g dried apples, chopped

1/2 tsp ground cinnamon (optional)

Directions

STEP 1

Heat the oven to 180C/160C fan/ gas 4. Butter the base of a 20 x 20cm square tin and line with baking parchment. Tip the chopped apples into a small saucepan with 2 tsp water and cook over a medium heat for 3-4 mins until the apples are just soft enough to crush, but there's still a little water left in the pan. If needed, add a little more water and cook the apples for slightly longer. Remove from the heat and crush the apples using a potato masher or a fork to break up slightly, then tip into a bowl and set aside.

STEP 2

Tip the butter, golden syrup and sugar into the pan and warm through over a low heat until the butter has melted and the sugar has dissolved. Remove from the heat and set aside.

STEP 3

Combine the oats, dried apple and cinnamon, if using, in a large bowl. Tip in the buttery syrup mix and cooked apples, then stir to combine. Tip the flapjack mixture into the prepared tin and press down firmly. Level the surface using a spatula, then bake for 25-30 mins until golden and bubbling at the sides. Leave to cool. Cut into 16 pieces. Will keep in an airtight container for three days.

Mini pumpkin & feta pies

Ingredients

450g butternut squash or pumpkin peeled and cut into 2cm chunks (prepared weight)

2 garlic cloves

2 tbsp olive oil

1 small onion, finely chopped

250g plain flour, plus extra for dusting

½ tsp ground turmeric

125g cold butter, cut into small pieces, plus extra for the tin

2 egg yolks plus 1 whole egg, beaten

grating of nutmeg

½ tsp chilli flakes (optional)

200g feta, crumbled

Directions

STEP 1

Heat the oven to 200C/180C fan/gas 6. Tip the squash and unpeeled garlic into a roasting tin, drizzle with 1 tbsp oil, season and toss to coat. Roast for 30 mins, stirring halfway through, until soft. Remove from the oven and leave to cool.

STEP 2

Meanwhile, cook the onion in a frying pan over a medium heat with the remaining 1 tbsp oil for 8-10 mins until tender and slightly golden. Leave to cool.

STEP 3

Tip the flour, turmeric and a pinch of salt into a food processor. Add the butter and whizz until the mixture resembles fine crumbs. Add the egg yolks and 2 tsp cold water, and blitz again until the mixture starts to clump together. Squeeze it between your fingers – if it sticks together, tip the mixture onto a work surface. If it's too dry, add more water, 1 tsp at a time. Knead the pastry a few times just to bring it together, but don't overwork it. Shape into two circles, one slightly smaller than the other, then wrap in baking parchment and chill in the fridge for at least 20 mins.

STEP 4

Squeeze the garlic from its skins into the roasted squash and mash together. Add the fried onion, grate over some nutmeg, tip in the chilli flakes, if using, and feta, and mix.

STEP 5

Butter six holes of a muffin tin and line each with a strip of baking parchment that overhangs the top. Roll the larger circle of pastry out on a lightly floured surface to the thickness of a £1 coin. Use a 10cm cutter to stamp out six circles (you may need to re-roll the pastry to get all six). Press the pastry circles into the prepared muffin tin, patching any cracks with the pastry offcuts. Spoon in the squash filling.

STEP 6

Roll the remaining pastry circle out as you did the large one, but use an 8cm cutter to cut out six lids. Cut spooky pumpkin faces into the lids using a small, sharp knife. Press the lids over the pies in the tin and brush with the beaten egg. Bake for 40 mins until golden brown, then leave to cool for 10 mins in the tin before lifting out. Eat hot or leave to cool completely. Will keep in an airtight container in the fridge for up to two days or the freezer for up to two months. Reheat in a low oven for 10 mins, if you like.

Classic guacamole

Ingredients

¼ red onion

2 ripe tomatoes

a few coriander sprigs

2 green jalapeños

2 ripe avocados, halved

1 lime, juiced

tortilla chips, to serve

Directions

STEP 1

Finely chop the red onion, tomatoes, coriander and jalapeños separately. Mix together the onion, tomatoes, coriander and a pinch of salt. Keep the jalapeños to one side.

STEP 2

Scoop all the avocado flesh into a bowl and crush with a fork, leaving it chunky – it should not be puréed. Add the lime juice and onion mixture, combining gently.

STEP 3

Add jalapeños, to taste, and more sea salt if needed. Serve with the tortilla chips.

Rhubarb & date chutney

Ingredients

50g fresh root ginger, grated

300ml red wine vinegar

500g eating apple, peeled and finely chopped

200g pitted date, chopped

200g dried cranberries or raisins

1 tbsp mustard seed

1 tbsp curry powder

400g light muscovado sugar

700g rhubarb, sliced into 2cm chunks

500g red onion

Directions

STEP 1

Put the onions in a large pan with the ginger and vinegar. Bring to the boil, then simmer for 10 mins. Add the rest of the Ingredients, except the rhubarb, plus 2 tsp salt to the pan and bring to the boil, stirring. Simmer, uncovered, for about 10 mins until the apples are tender.

STEP 2

Stir in the rhubarb and cook, uncovered, until the chutney is thick and jammy, about 15-20 mins. Leave the chutney to sit for about 10-15 mins, then spoon into warm, clean jars, and seal. Label the jars when cool. Keep for at least a month before eating.

Cheese & rosemary biscuits

Ingredients

80g wholemeal flour

80g plain flour

100g cold butter, chopped

100g cheddar, finely grated

1 small rosemary sprig, leaves finely chopped

1 large egg yolk

Directions

STEP 1

Heat oven to 180C/160C fan/ gas 4. Put the flours in a bowl and rub in the butter until it resembles breadcrumbs. Stir in the cheese and rosemary, then add the yolk and mix in using a fork. When the mix starts to clump together, use your hands to knead to a smooth dough.

STEP 2

Take walnut-sized pieces of dough, roll into balls and place on one or two lined baking trays. Flatten slightly with a fork, then bake for 12-14 mins. Alternatively, roll out between sheets of baking parchment and cut into shapes, then bake as before. Cool on the baking sheet for a few mins before moving to a wire rack to cool completely. Store in an airtight container for up to a week.

Air-fryer soy & cranberry chicken wings

Ingredients

1kg chicken wings

3 tbsp soy sauce

6 tbsp cranberry sauce

1 tsp dried oregano

2 garlic cloves, crushed

2 tsp ginger paste or freshly grated ginger

2 tsp vegetable oil

Directions

STEP 1

Pat the chicken wings dry using a clean tea towel or kitchen paper (this helps ensure the wings crisp up). Heat the air-fryer to 200C. Combine the soy sauce, cranberry sauce, oregano, garlic, ginger and vegetable oil in a small bowl or jug. Put the chicken wings in a large bowl, then spoon or pour over the cranberry mixture.

STEP 2

Toss everything together and mix well so the chicken wings are well coated. The uncooked wings will keep frozen in an airtight container for up to three months. Tip the wings into the air-fryer basket and cook for 15-20 mins at 200C (or 20-25 mins at 180C from frozen), turning halfway through until cooked through and beginning to brown at the edges. You may need to do this in two batches depending on the size of your air-fryer.

Halloumi fries

Ingredients

170g pot Greek yogurt

1 lemon, zested, then cut into wedges for squeezing

1 tbsp rose harissa

3 tbsp za'atar, plus extra for sprinkling

75g plain flour

2 x 250g blocks halloumi, cut into fries

oil, for frying

handful mint, leaves torn

Directions

STEP 1

Mix the yogurt with the lemon zest and some seasoning, then swirl through the harissa so that you have pockets of hot and cool in the dip.

STEP 2

On a plate, stir the za'atar into the flour, then roll the halloumi in the mixture so that it's evenly coated. Heat the oil in a shallow, heavy-bottomed pan or casserole dish until 180C on a cooking thermometer, or a piece of bread browns in 20 secs. Working in batches, carefully lower the halloumi into the oil and cook for 2 mins until crisp and golden, then drain on kitchen paper.

STEP 3

Sprinkle over the mint and za'atar, and serve with the lemon wedges and the spicy yogurt for dipping.

Malt loaf

Ingredients

sunflower oil, for greasing

150ml hot black tea

175g malt extract, plus extra for glazing (see tip)

85g dark muscovado sugar

300g mixed dried fruit

2 large eggs, beaten

250g plain flour

1 tsp baking powder

½ tsp bicarbonate of soda

Directions

STEP 1

Heat oven to 150C/130C fan/gas 2. Line the base and ends of two greased 450g/1lb non-stick loaf tins with strips of baking parchment.

STEP 2

Pour the hot tea into a mixing bowl with the malt, sugar and dried fruit. Stir well, then add the eggs.

STEP 3

Tip in the flour, then quickly stir in the baking powder and bicarbonate of soda and pour into the prepared tins. Bake for 50 mins until firm and well risen. While still warm, brush with a little more malt to glaze and leave to cool.

STEP 4

Remove from the tins. If you can bear not to eat it straight away, it gets more sticky after wrapping and keeping for 2-5 days. Serve sliced and buttered, if you like.

Egg & rocket pizzas

Ingredients

2 seeded wraps

a little olive oil, for brushing

1 roasted red pepper, from a jar

2 tomatoes

2 tbsp tomato purée

1 tbsp chopped dill

2 tbsp chopped parsley

2 eggs

65g pack rocket

½ red onion, very thinly sliced

Directions

STEP 1

Heat oven to 200C/180C fan/gas 6. Lay the tortillas on two baking sheets, brush sparingly with the oil then bake for 3 mins. Meanwhile chop the pepper and tomatoes and mix with the tomato purée, seasoning and herbs. Turn the tortillas over and spread with the tomato mixture, leaving the centre free from any large pieces of pepper or tomato.

STEP 2

Break an egg into the centre then return to the oven for 10 mins or until the egg is just set and the tortilla is crispy round the edges. Serve scattered with the rocket and onion.

Leek, bacon & mustard quesadilla

Ingredients

1 tbsp butter

1 large leek, sliced

3 smoked streaky bacon rashers, chopped

1 tbsp wholegrain mustard

1 tbsp chopped parsley

30g mature cheddar, grated

30g mozzarella, grated

2 large flour tortillas

Directions

STEP 1

Heat the butter in a small frying pan set over a medium heat. Fry the leek for 10 mins until softened. Transfer to a bowl and leave to cool for 15 mins. Fry the bacon in the pan for 5 mins, or until crisp. Mix the leeks with the mustard, parsley, cheddar and mozzarella. Spread the mixture over 1 tortilla and top with the bacon and second tortilla.

STEP 2

Heat a frying pan over a high heat. When hot, add the quesadilla and cook for 2 mins on one side. Turn it over and cook for 1-2 mins more, or until the cheese is melted. Cut into four.

CHAPTER FIVE

JUST ONE FINAL THING TO ADDRESS BEFORE YOU GO!

After delving into the available research on interstitial cystitis and its association with diet, it seems evident that dietary adjustments could hold significance in symptom management for some individuals. While there's no universal formula, evidence indicates that steering clear of certain trigger foods like acidic fruits, caffeine, alcohol, and spicy dishes, while incorporating bladder-friendly options such as water-rich vegetables, lean proteins, and whole grains, might offer relief and enhance overall well-being. However, it's crucial for those dealing with interstitial cystitis to find a supportive health care provider who is concerned about your quality of life as well as someone who will work with you to help relieve your urinary frequency, urgency and bladder pain.

Support from family and friends is important, but because the condition is a urinary problem, you may find the topic difficult to discuss.

Alternatively, you might benefit from joining a support group. A support group can provide sympathetic listening and useful information. Ask your provider for information on support groups or see the Interstitial Cystitis Association on the web.

9 798327 068049